Connecting Through the Heart

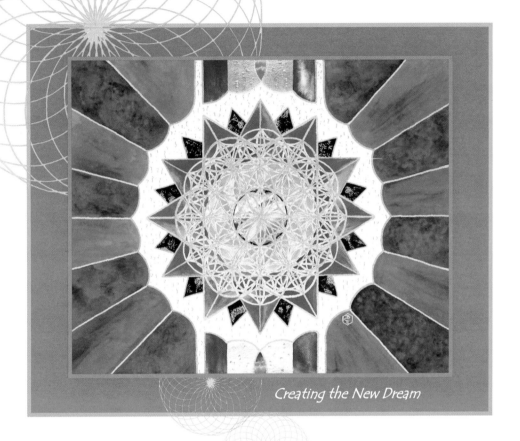

Creating the New Dream

Belongs to ....

The Journey begins ....

Healing Vibrations

Awaken my Heart and Soul

Inspiring New Life

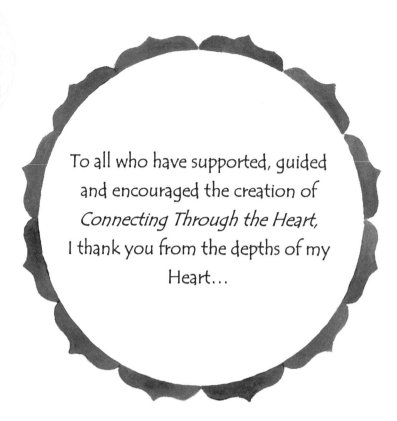

To all who have supported, guided
and encouraged the creation of
Connecting Through the Heart,
I thank you from the depths of my
Heart...

Published by Crystal Wings Healing Art. All rights reserved.

No part of this Journal may be used or reproduced in any manner for private or public use, other than brief quotations embodied in articles or reviews, without prior written permission from the publisher.

Crystal Wings Healing Art LLC, Richland MI 49083

(269) 731 2649

www.CrystalWingsHealingArt.com

All artwork and cover design by Barbara Evans

ISBN 978-0-9836369-3-9

This Mandala Coloring Journal provides support for spiritual growth and wellbeing.
It does not replace medical or psychological diagnosis, counseling and treatment.

Welcome

Twenty years ago I began a journey to find a new way of living and being within the world... a way that invites and enhances wellbeing on all levels of Body, Mind and Spirit.

I discovered within myself a gift of translating positive frequencies such as Love, Hope and Joy, that support all aspects of our health at a very deep level, into art. I call this art, Transformational Healing Art.

Transformational Healing Art helps us to raise our consciousness, shifting our perspective from negative vibrations of anxiety, fear and isolation, to positive feelings of Connectedness, Hope, Joy and Harmony. Raising our consciousness creates a positive impact on all aspects of our lives, including physical wellness.

Within, you will find ten mandala coloring templates, inspiring paintings, positive messages, and plenty of pages for your own journaling and creative expression.

My intention is for this Mandala Coloring Journal to support you, as you set out on a journey to activate more of your own inner healing abilities and bring them into your daily life experience. Coloring the mandala templates helps this process to unfold effortlessly, assisting you to connect with the inner beauty that lies deep within your heart.

With Love and Blessings

Barbara Evans

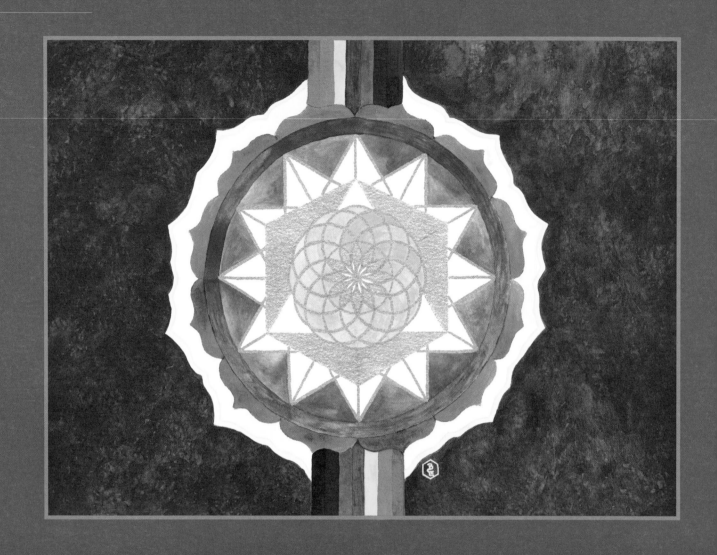

Healing ... Emotions

As you prepare to color your mandala... Imagine...
Waves of Love gently washing away emotional wounds held
deep within your Heart... Feel your Heart begin to open,
heal and overflow with these waves of Love.

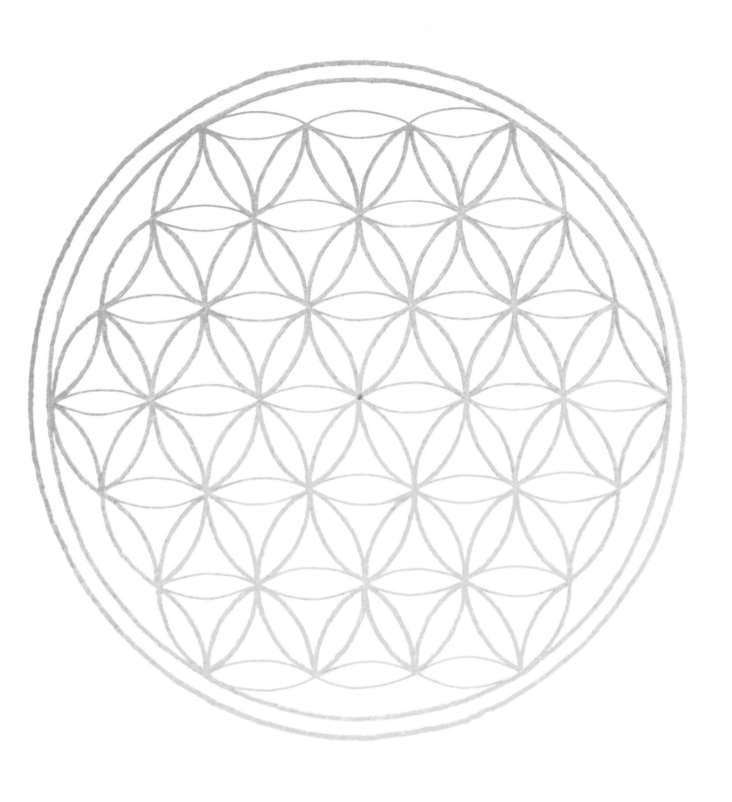

Connecting Through the Heart: Mandala 1

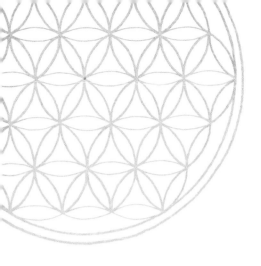
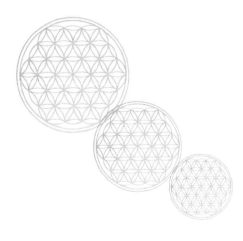

As my heart fills with LOVE...

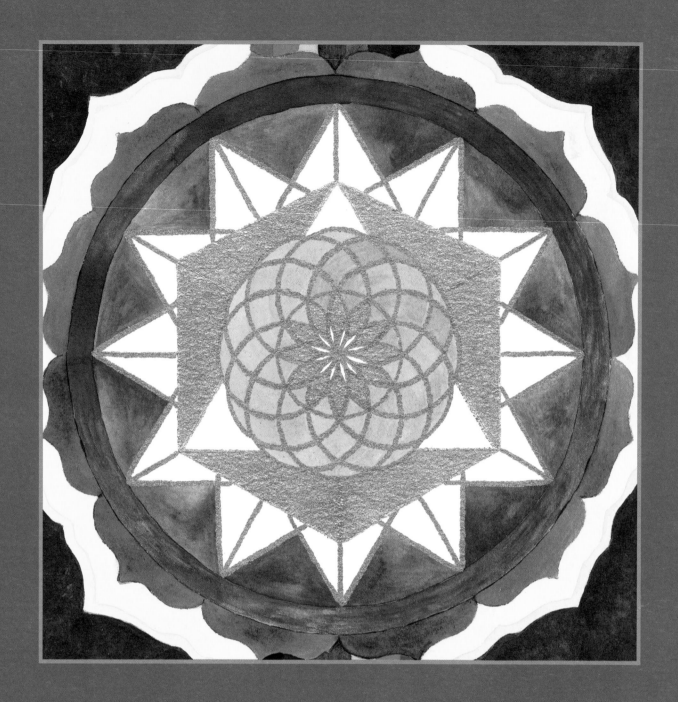

Healing ...Thoughts

As you prepare to color your mandala... Imagine...

**A gentle breeze blows through your Mind,
replacing negative thoughts and fears with inspiring
thoughts of Peace, Contentment and Healing.**

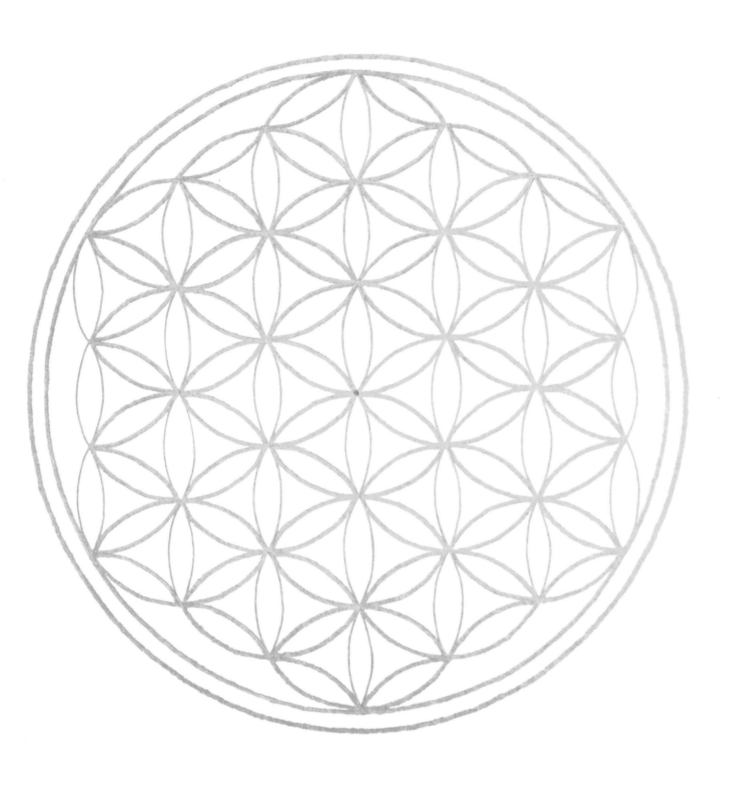

Connecting Through the Heart: Mandala 2

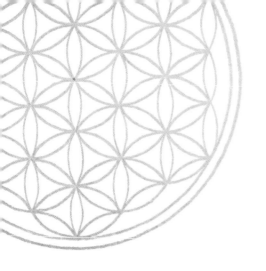

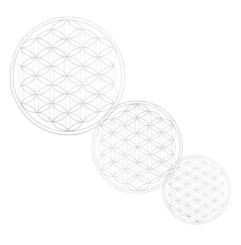

As my mind fills with Healing Thoughts...

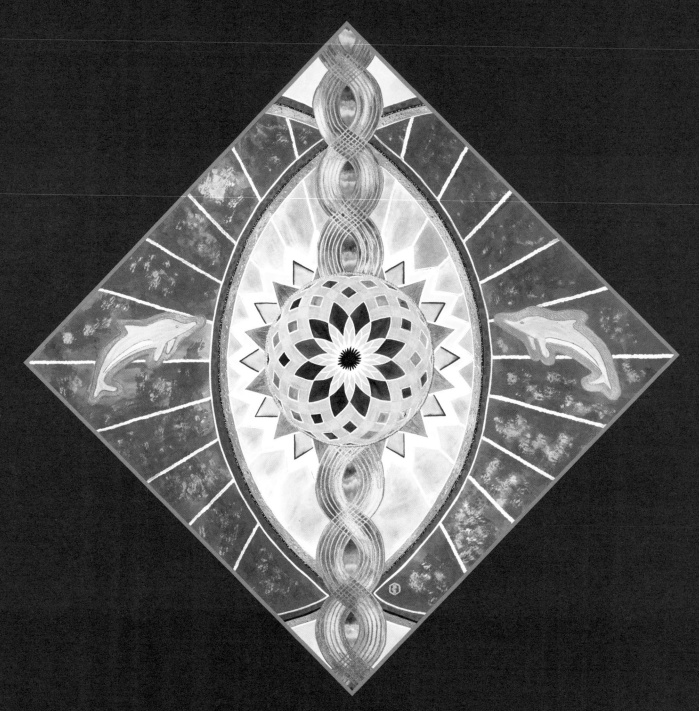

Awakening Creativity

As you prepare to color your next mandala... Consider...

Creativity is an important foundation of vitality, health
and well-being. Coloring this mandala encourages you
to connect with your Creative side...

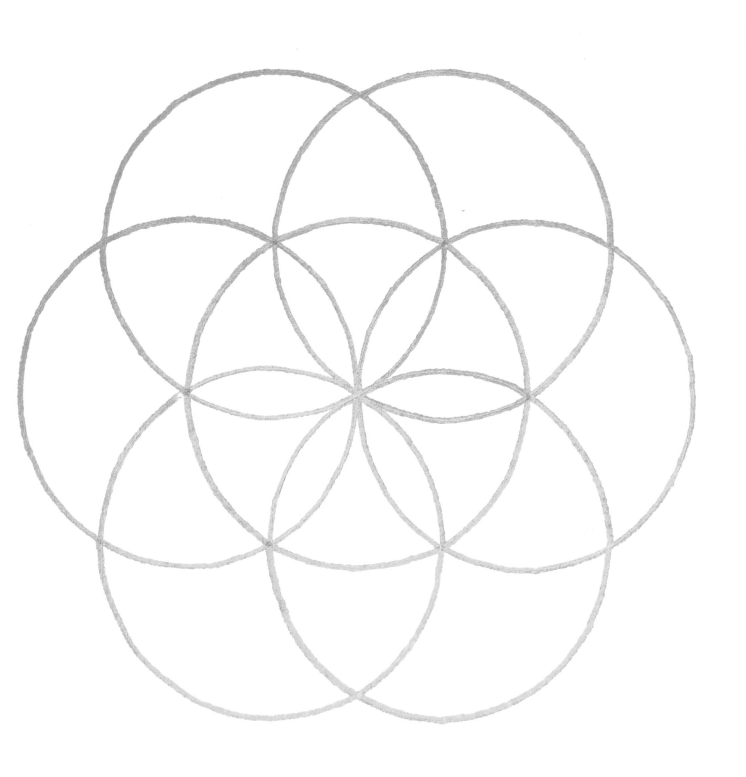

Connecting Through the Heart: Mandala 3

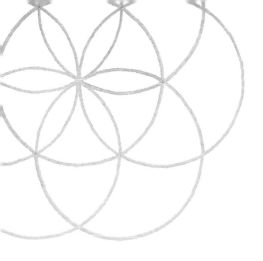

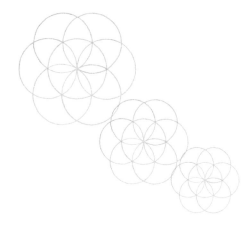

New Creative Ideas are...

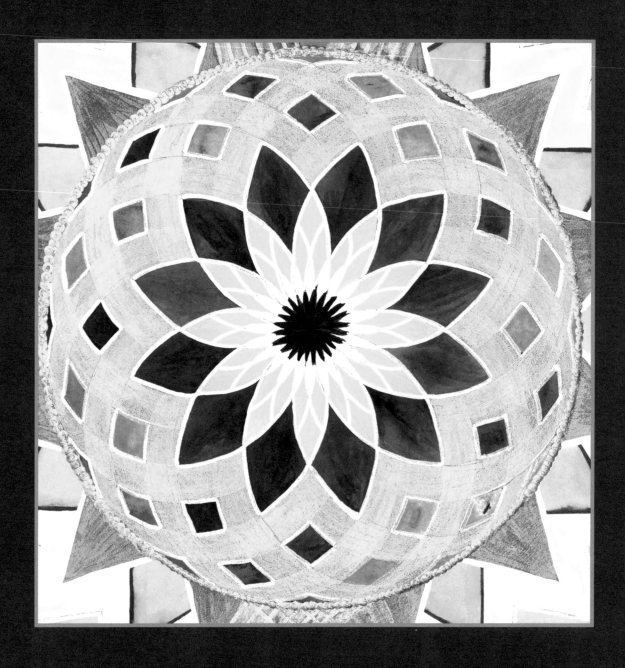

Awakening Wisdom

As you prepare to color your next mandala... Consider...

Wisdom emerges through integrating life experiences with clarity of thought. Coloring this mandala encourages you to connect with your innate Inner Wisdom...

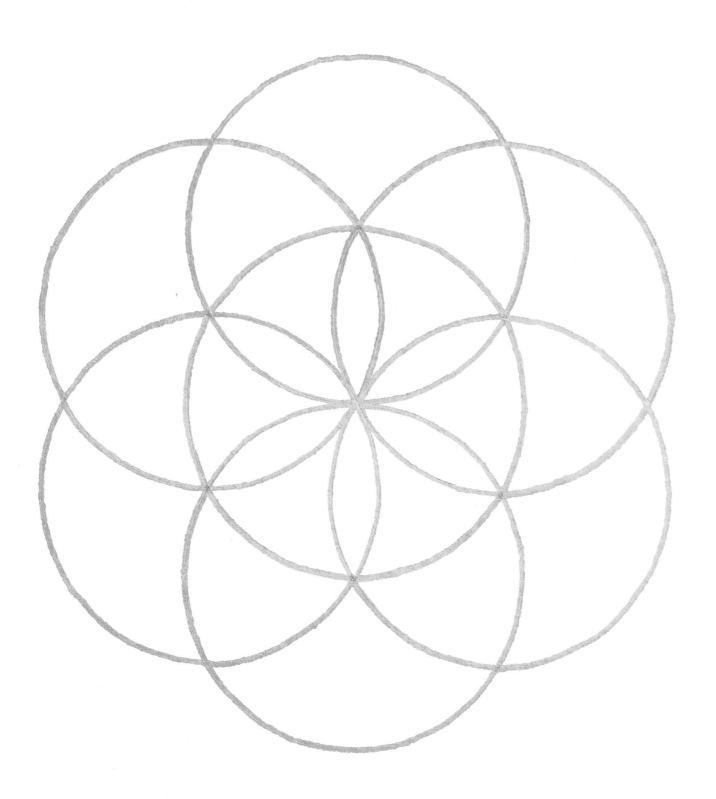

Connecting Through the Heart: Mandala 4

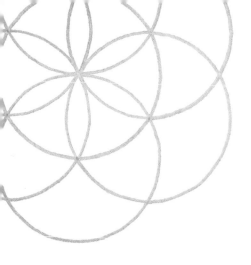

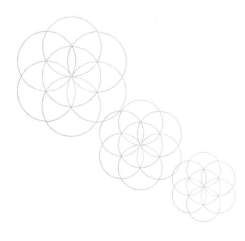

I acknowledge my Inner Wisdom...

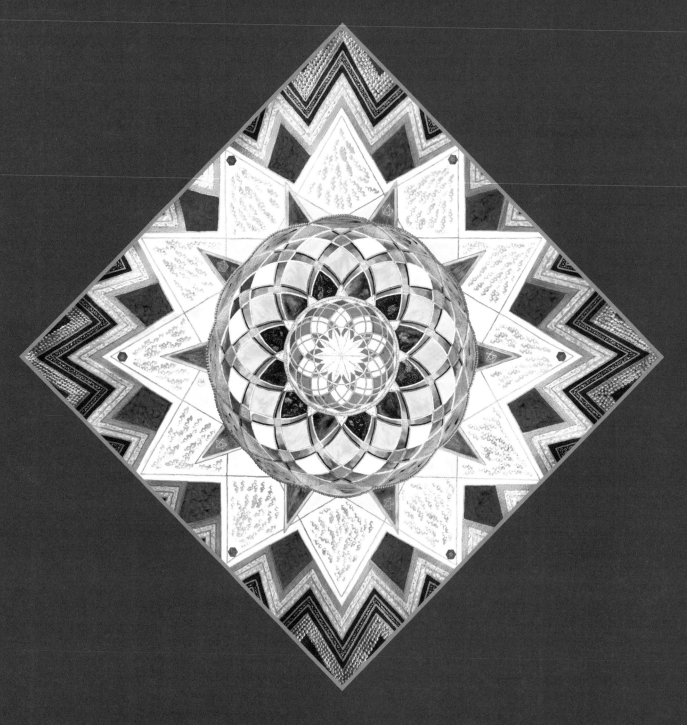

Hope

As you prepare to color your next mandala...

Hope is like a spark of Love connecting Heart and Soul.
Imagine ...Hope blossoming deep within every cell, ready
to inspire new life ...

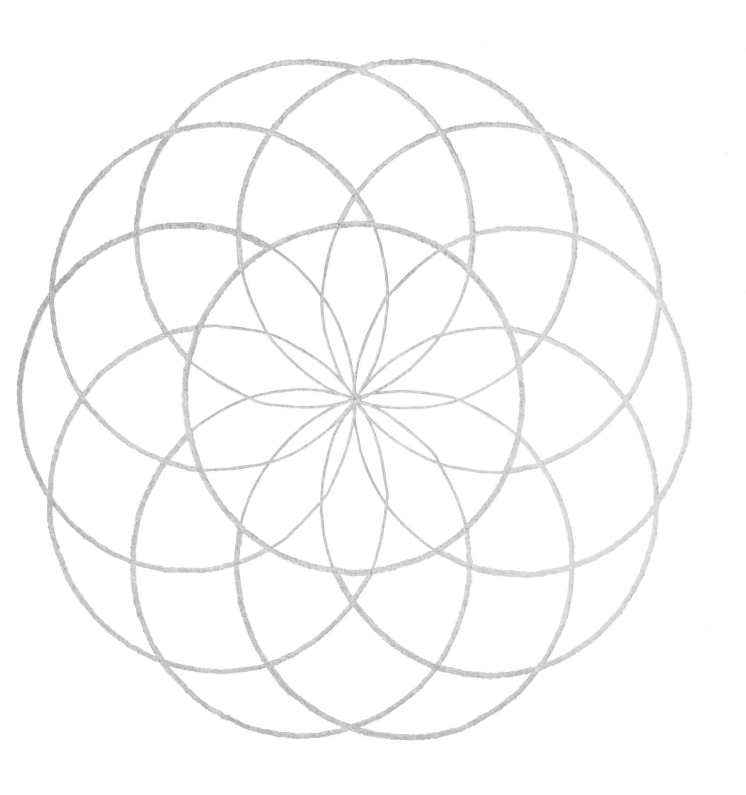

Connecting Through the Heart: Mandala 5

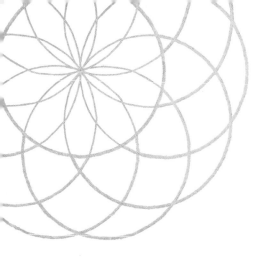

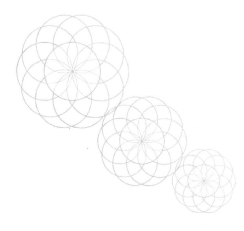

I Hope...

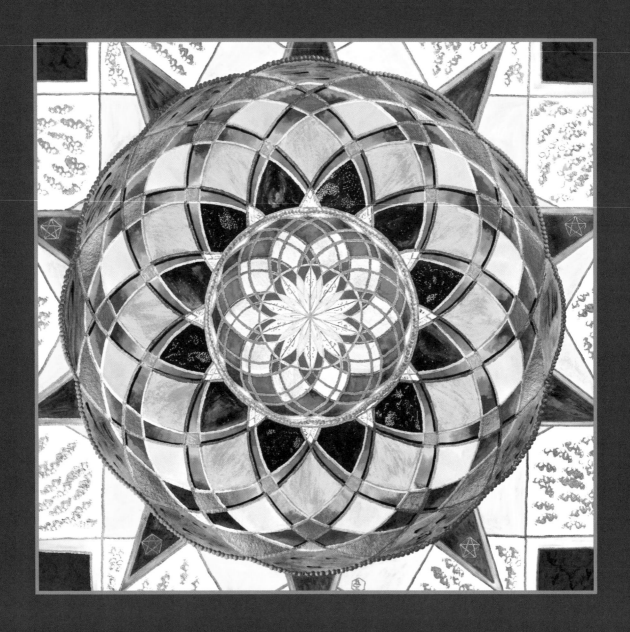

Dream

As you prepare to color your next mandala...

Imagine a beautiful dream that fills you with Hope...

As you color, allow these positive emotions to permeate every cell of your being.

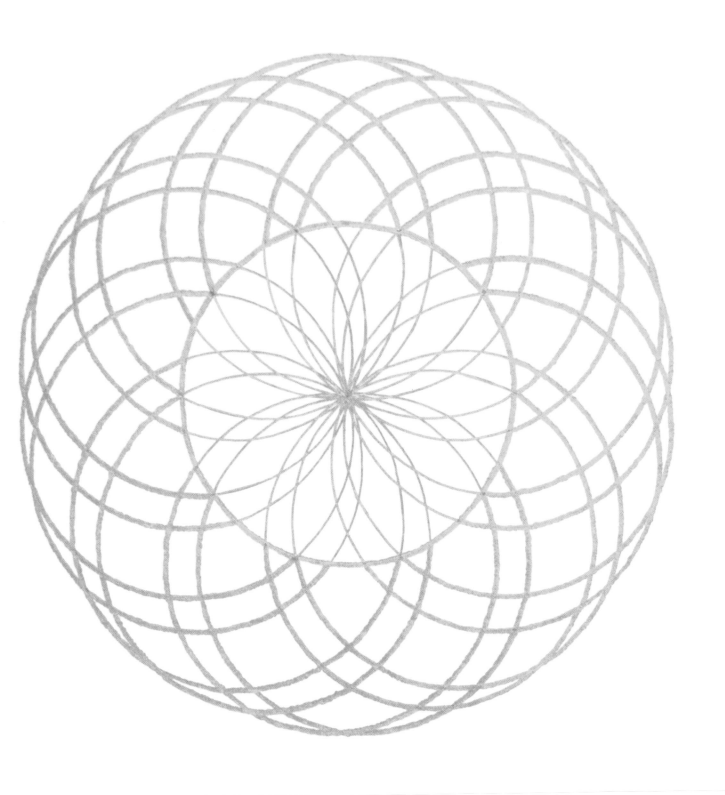

Connecting Through the Heart: Mandala 6

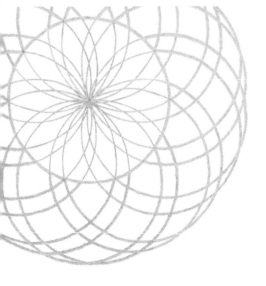

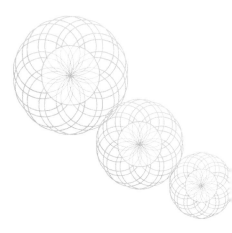

My Dreams inspire...

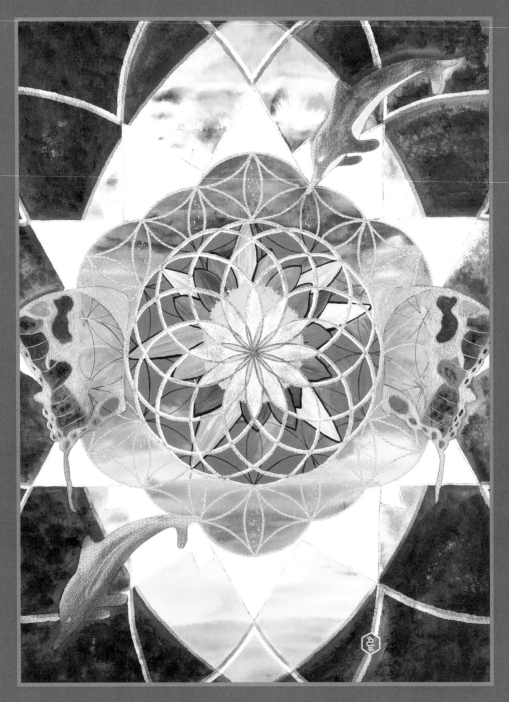

Transformation

As you prepare to color your next mandala...   Consider...

Transformation comes from shifting your perspective and focusing on positive thoughts and emotions... this mandala helps you transform to a place of Balance and Harmony.

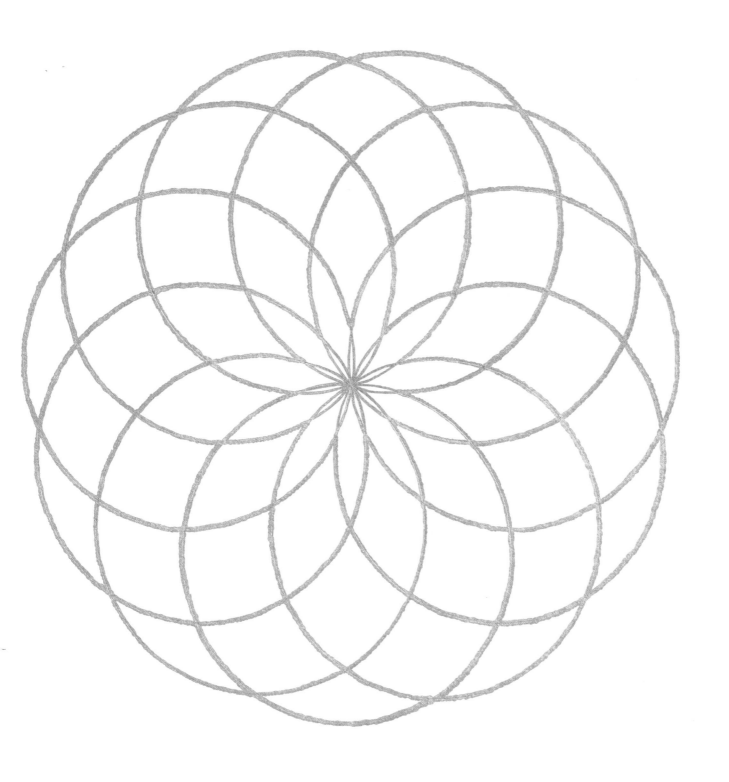

Connecting Through the Heart: Mandala 7

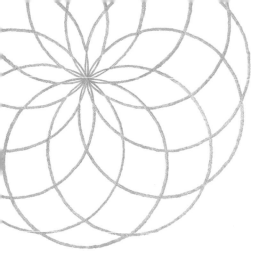

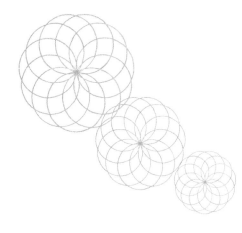

Transformation means...

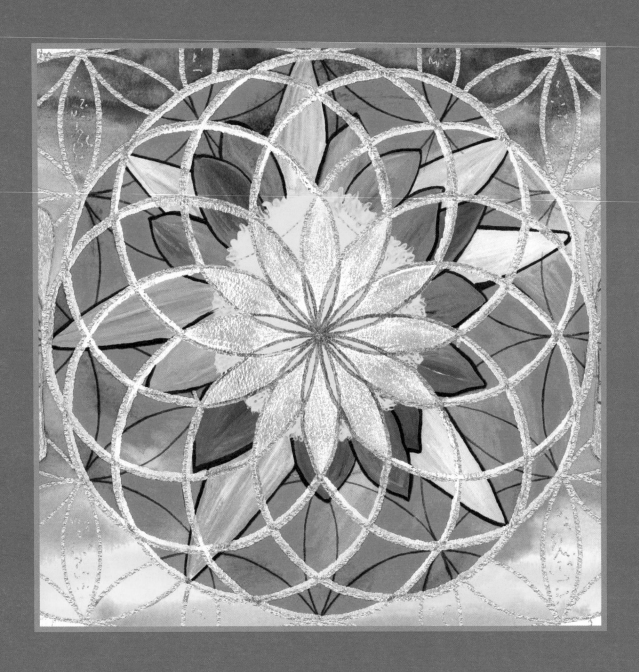

Gateway

As you prepare to color the next picture... Consider...

This mandala is like a Gateway to higher consciousness... offering an opportunity to infuse your life with a heightened sense of Peace and Joy...

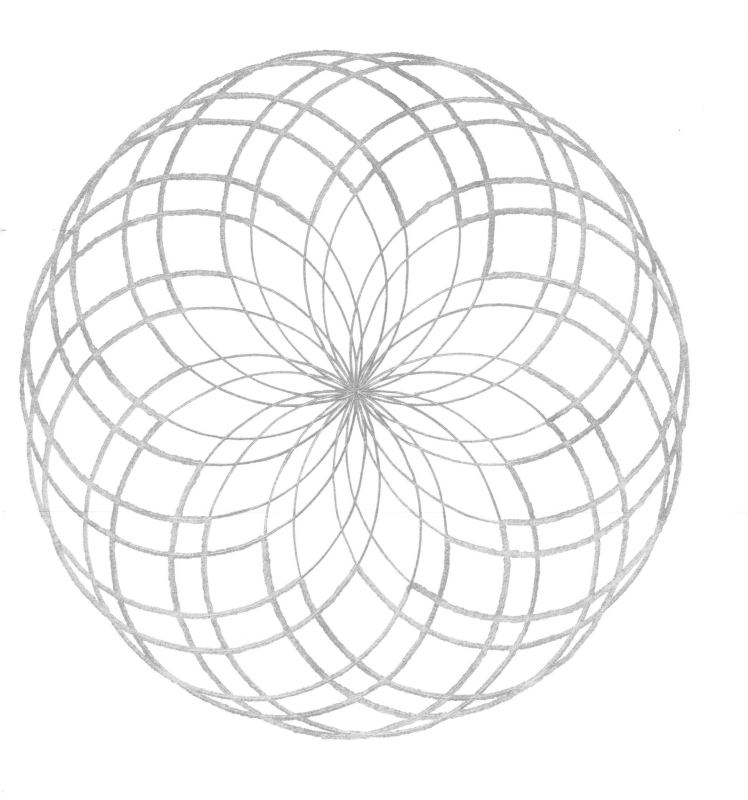

Connecting Through the Heart: Mandala 8

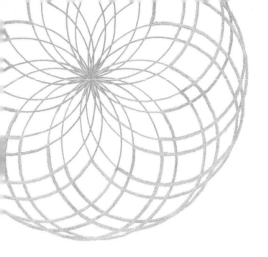

As I step through the gateway...

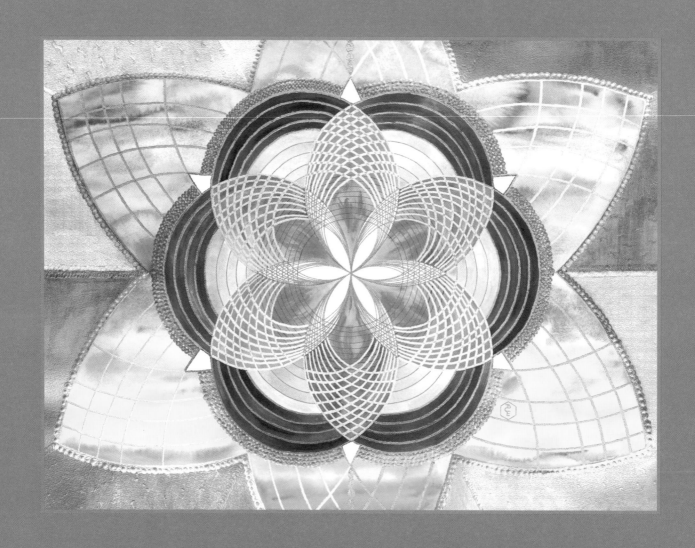

Abundance...

As you prepare to color the next mandala... Imagine...

Like a sunrise ... this mandala immerses you in an abundance of life giving energy, expanding awareness of your true Self or Essence ...

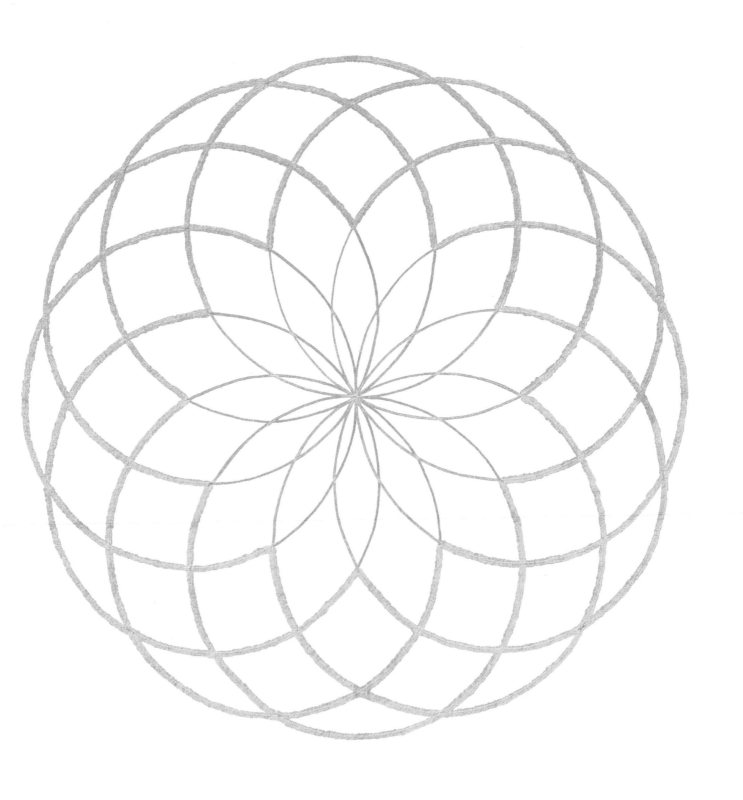

Connecting Through the Heart: Mandala 9

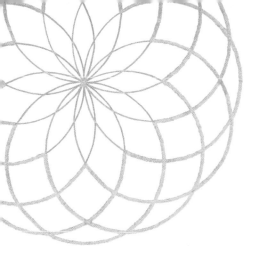

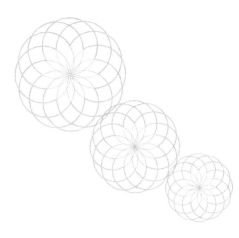

My true Essence...

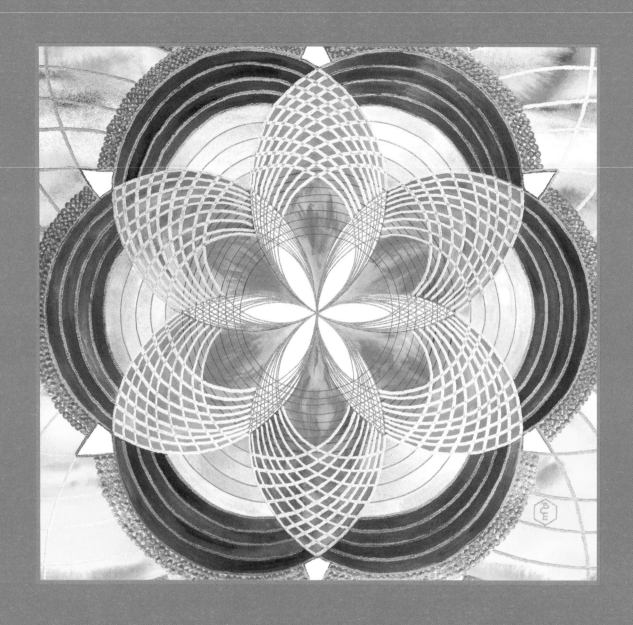

Possibilities...

As you prepare to color this final mandala... Imagine...

All Possibilities are Open with no limitations ... Connect with the feelings deep within your Heart that yearn to be expressed, and the inspiring thoughts within your Mind that call to be heard...

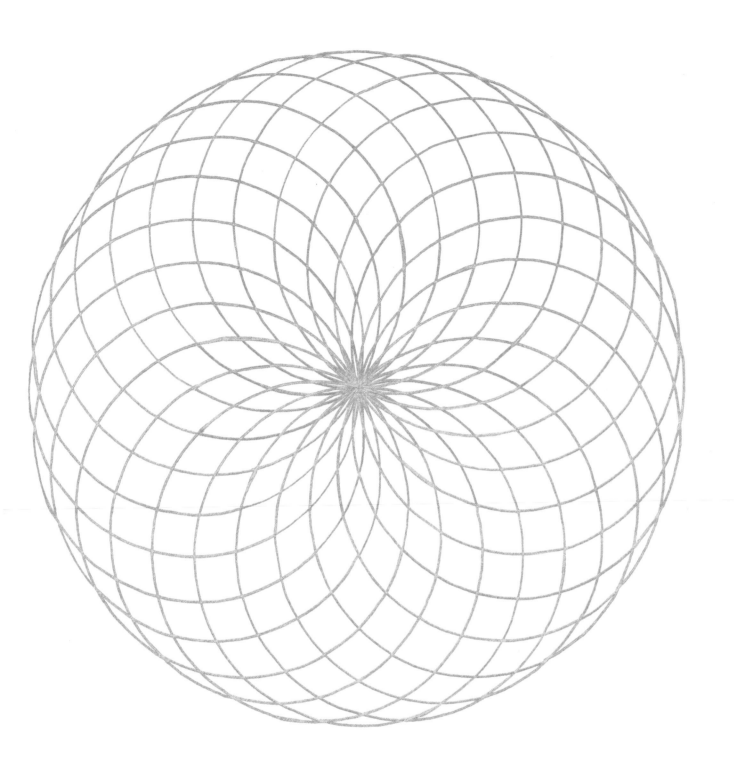

Connecting Through the Heart: Mandala 10

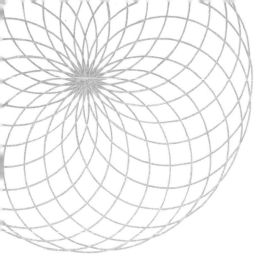

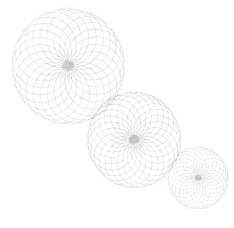

I really wish...

A New Journey Has Begun ...

I hope that you have enjoyed creating your own, very personal, journey of *Connecting Through the Heart*, and that the experience has offered many blessings, helping you feel the energy of Universal Love as it surrounds, warms and supports you!

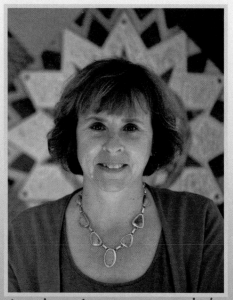

Barbara Evans is an award winning author and transformational healing artist, whose book, *Messages of Universal Wisdom* and beautiful *Image Key* paintings have gained international recognition. The *Image Keys* radiate vibrations which contribute to healing via the raising of consciousness and connection to our Inner Essence. Barbara's artwork is now the foundation of a new energy healing approach, *The Eden Method.™*

From the beginning of her career as an artist, Barbara has held an inner mission to enhance patient experience within our Healthcare System. Her broader vision is to help Create a New Earth and New Dream based upon Peace, Beauty and Joy.

Barbara@CrystalWingsHealingArt.com

Further information is available at: www.CrystalWingsHealingArt.com